Living Young Forever

The Secret Formula to Longevity and Good Health.

By

Dr. Benjamin N. Nunn

Copyright

Table of content

About the Book

Growing old and looking aged and fragile was once considered a normal occurrence. We believe that illness, weakness, and progressive aging are unavoidable aspects of our existence. Yet they are not required to be so. Today's science views aging as an illness that can be remedied. We may extend our healthy lives and cure age-related diseases such as dementia, diabetes, cancer, and heart disease by treating the core causes of these conditions.

Dr. Benjamin N. Nunn encourages us to rethink our biology, health, and the aging process in Living Young Forever. He examines the biological signs of aging, their origins, and their effects to discover the keys to longevity. He then demonstrates how to combat these biological signs of age using straightforward nutritional, lifestyle, and newly discovered longevity techniques. You'll discover:
The key to activating your switch for longevity
Therapy for Inflammation: 3 Immune System Calming Techniques

How to get enough sleep, exercise, and relax for healthy aging
How to eat well balance diet for a long life
Choosing the appropriate supplements for you
Where the future of aging research is going
And a lot more
Living Young Forever is a ground-breaking practical guide to achieving and maintaining health—for life—with hundreds of science-based techniques and suggestions.

Chapter 1.

The key to activating your switch for longevity

The capacity of an antioxidant to support people living longer, healthier lives is gaining increasing attention these days. This antioxidant is well-known to researchers but not to the general population.

Because of its capacity to strengthen certain genes that are essential for surviving well into your elderly years, this antioxidant is like a switch for longevity that may extend life. This may be one of the most effective antioxidant/anti-inflammatory combos to have been found lately.

I'll also explain how to "turn the switch" right after. But first, let's discuss these research results in greater detail.

A recent, possibly ground-breaking examination of an antioxidant that isn't exactly well-known (which is presumably why it didn't get much public attention) may hold the key to finding the solution. I'm referencing astaxanthin.

So don't let the lack of information about the potency of this drug mislead you.

The findings' importance might change everything for you or any person who desires to live a long, healthy life.

Activating the gene for long life

Astaxanthin has an antioxidant capacity that is 6,000 times more than that of vitamin C and 800 times greater than that of CoQ10.

And in terms of the incredible health advantages of this substance, it is only the tip of the iceberg. Astaxanthin also aids in reducing:

- Triglycerides
- Inflammation
- liver injury
- heart injury
- stroke danger

The chance of developing heart disease, dementia, arthritis, and visual issues is decreased by all of these advantages.

The switch for longevity is another factor that I mentioned previously. This is based on how astaxanthin influences the FOXO3 gene. You are protected by several aging factors thanks to this gene.

A research project conducted by the University of Hawaii academics set out to look into this. Three different diets—normal, low, and high in astaxanthin—were given to the mice.

An analysis of cardiac tissue revealed that a high astaxanthin diet significantly increased FOXO3 gene activity. The JABSOM team is certain that further human studies will provide comparable outcomes. The effects of astaxanthin on cognitive performance in people with early dementia are already being studied in humans, and more animal studies are also being carried out.

Even if it may be too soon to start rejoicing over the discovery of the secret of youthfulness, it's never too early to start taking astaxanthin tablets.

The color of long-lasting health

Astaxanthin is a deep yellow-orange-red chemical that is present in kelp, fish, shrimp, and other crustaceans. Moreover, it is prevalent in turmeric, which is the healthiest spice in your kitchen, sweet potatoes, and leafy green vegetables.

At the molecular level, astaxanthin guards you against aging in several unique ways. Only three of them are briefly highlighted below:

a. Since it protects both the lipid-soluble and water-soluble components of the cell, astaxanthin provides whole cellular protection.

b. Being one of the few nutrients that can pass the blood-brain barrier, astaxanthin protects the brain's sensitive neurons against oxidative damage.

c. Astaxanthin guards against DNA deterioration and protects mitochondria, the "energy factories" that give each cell its power.

Since it's difficult to get sufficient amounts from diet alone, it's crucial to supplement with astaxanthin. To receive a minimum daily intake, for instance, you would need to consume around one pound of salmon every day.

Consequently, it is advised to take 4 to 16 milligrams of astaxanthin daily in addition to the dietary sources I stated before. So, be cautious while picking an astaxanthin supplement. The supply from natural marine sources has not been able to keep up with the

rise in demand for this carotenoid. While the
market is overrun with synthetic alternatives,
natural sources are still accessible

CHAPTER 2

Therapy for Inflammation: 3 Immune System Calming Techniques

This chapter will teach you how to manage inflammation both internal and external by combining medicine, diet, and stress reduction approaches.

The relationship between inflammation and a wide range of illnesses and medical issues has also been uncovered as medical professionals understand more about inflammation and how it impacts our general health.

As inflammation affects almost every organ in the body, including the heart, lungs, bones, joints, skin, brain, and more, physicians often advise a multifaceted treatment plan for it.

While inflammation is sometimes associated with negative connotations, it is your immune system's method of developing a defense against viruses or bacteria or aiding the healing and protection of a wounded part of the body by boosting blood flow there. This reaction serves to protect us from trauma.

But, inflammation may turn harmful to your health if it becomes a persistent, systemic condition.

Inflammation: Its Causes and Forms

Many factors, including an infection, a physical injury, or an overactive immune system, may promote inflammation. The triggers lead to swelling of the arteries, which increases blood flow to the wounded area, the accumulation of fluid and proteins, and the release of a kind of white blood cell known as a neutrophil by the body. When these three things happen, inflammatory symptoms start to show themselves.

There are two types of inflammation: acute and chronic. Acute inflammation symptoms develop rapidly, may become severe fast, and are often alleviated with therapy within a few days or weeks.

Acute inflammation may be brought on by the following conditions:

Meningitis

- Sinusitis\sDermatitis
- Bronchitis\sTonsillitis\sAppendicitis
- a physical harm

- cold or flu-related sore throat
- scrapes, burns, or cuts
- Exercise

Long-term inflammation may linger for months or even years. It may happen due to an autoimmune illness in some situations or acute inflammation that was left untreated in others. Chronic inflammation may result from the following conditions:

- inflammatory colitis
- Crohn's illness
- arthritis rheumatoid
- Sinusitis
- Hepatitis
- stomach ulcer
- Periodontitis
- Tuberculosis
- Asthma

Many age-related disorders, such as metabolic syndrome, diabetes, heart disease, cancer, dementia, and osteoporosis have been linked to chronic inflammation.

Tests and Signs of Inflammation

The signs of acute inflammation are extremely obvious.

These may result in discomfort, bruising, redness, and loss of function in the afflicted area of the body and skin.

Yet, chronic inflammation often goes undiagnosed or is misinterpreted for other illnesses. Some symptoms include:

- Continual tiredness
- Constipation, diarrhea, bloating, and other digestive problems
- gaining weight
- elevated blood pressure
- Acne
- aching joints
- Skin blotchiness or rashes

Evaluation of Inflammation

Doctors employ a variety of blood tests to identify both acute and chronic inflammation. High sensitivity C-reactive Protein (hs-CRP), the most popular test, measures a protein the body produces in reaction to inflammation.

This examination is excellent for identifying low-grade, persistent, and systemic inflammation and is very accurate in estimating your risk of suffering a heart attack or stroke. Fasting insulin, hemoglobin A1c, serum ferritin, and red blood cell counts are further examinations physicians employ to gauge inflammation in the body.

Three Popular Remedies for Inflammation

Your doctor may advise one or more of the following inflammatory therapies to treat or control the problem that's causing it, depending on the kind and degree of inflammation present inside the body.

1. **Medicine**

NSAIDs, also known as nonsteroidal anti-inflammatory medicines, are often used to treat headaches, muscular discomfort, and arthritis-related inflammation. Ibuprofen, naproxen, and celecoxib are some of the most popular NSAIDs that physicians advise patients to use.

Corticosteroids, a class of steroid hormones that contains cortisol, are broken down into two smaller classes: glucocorticoids and mineralocorticoids, which are both used to treat Addison's illness and cerebral salt wasting as well as arthritis, lupus, IBS, and arthritis.
drugs that fight viruses and antibiotics. Your doctor could advise antibiotics if tests show that a bacterial infection is the root of your inflammation. Several medicines, including penicillin, are sometimes used to treat gastric ulcers, sinusitis, periodontitis, meningitis, and periodontitis. Your doctor may recommend antiviral drugs for illnesses like the flu and hepatitis if inflammation is present as a result of a viral infection. While these medications cannot destroy viruses, they may stop them from growing.
According to the Arthritis Foundation, disease-modifying antirheumatic medicines (DMARDs) protect joints by reducing inflammation.

A unique class of DMARD called biologics is intended to halt joint deterioration and decrease inflammation.

According to a 2019 publication in the Frontiers in Psychiatry Journal, statins reduce LDL cholesterol, which has anti-inflammatory benefits.

2. **Nutrition**

Your chronic inflammation may be cured or fed by the foods you consume. Vitamin K, antioxidants, and omega-3 fatty acids should all be abundant in your diet since they may reduce inflammation. You should thus consume a lot of fruits, leafy green vegetables, nuts, seeds, and seafood. Trans fats, fried meals, and excessive quantities of fatty meat should be avoided since they may have the opposite impact.

Moreover, certain herbs and spices may be added to meals and drinks or taken as supplements and are recognized by medical professionals as anti-inflammatory therapy. These include:

- Turmeric
- Ginger
- Cinnamon

- Chili pepper
- Chilies
- Garlic
- Clove
- roasted pepper

3. **Decreased tension**

According to many experts, maintaining low levels of stress via regular exercise, sound sleep habits, and stress reduction practices is the key to avoiding inflammation.

Inflammation of the low-grade kind, which may result in chronic tiredness, obesity, and other significant disorders, can be treated with stress reduction. Many studies have linked inflammation, weariness, and stress.

Researchers found that stress may prevent the body from using the hormone cortisol to control inflammation. The hormone cortisol helps to manage inflammation in part, and when cortisol isn't permitted to do its job, inflammation may spiral out of control.

If you have persistent anxiety, let your doctor know and make an effort to reduce the stress in your life.

You may want to think about stress-relieving practices like mindfulness or meditation, or you might pick an activity you like that can help you forget about your troubles.

Chapter 3

The Role of Exercise in Preventing Aging
Everyone is aware of the health benefits of exercise, it helps everyone, not just the young, healthy, and physically fit. It is among the finest barriers against the most challenging parts of becoming older.

In addition to enhancing heart and lung health, research demonstrates that even a little exercise is beneficial to the brain, bones, muscles, and mood. Lifelong exercise may help individuals stay healthy for longer, prevent the start of 40 chronic disorders or diseases, prevent cognitive decline, lower their chance of falling, decrease their stress levels, and even extend their life. Exercise is our greatest line of defense and repairs against the many aging-related factors. There is strong evidence that exercise may stimulate the mechanisms required for DNA repair, however, it cannot of itself reverse aging. Of course, it is best to start exercising as soon as possible and keep doing so for as long as possible.

Yet, it is crucial to be active at any age.

There have been gains in the physical, cognitive, and mental health of nursing home patients, from research, carried out on the subject.

Note that while your risk for Alzheimer's disease, cardiovascular disease, Type 2 diabetes, cancer, or other aging-related disorders may not significantly rise until middle age or later, the underlying biology for such conditions is already in action from a young age. That trajectory is predetermined by your genetics and the lifestyle choices you make, but they may affect your risk for illness at any time. Hence, the phrase "too little, too late" is untrue. The good news is that you may benefit from exercise's anti-aging properties without signing up for a marathon or joining a gym. As long as it is done frequently, even a little physical exercise, such as walking the dog or choosing the stairs over the elevator, has positive effects on the body, soul, and spirit. These are just a few ways that regular action improves your health.

1. It increases muscular strength.

Sarcopenia is a disorder in which individuals lose muscle mass and strength as they age. Resistance exercise is one of the greatest strategies, according to scientists, to halt that decrease. It keeps your muscles strong, which you'll need to open jars and push heavy doors, and it also makes daily tasks like cooking, cleaning, and climbing stairs easier. Also, it may lessen your vulnerability to illness, enhance your mood and cognitive health, and support extended periods of independence. Resistance training is safe and beneficial for older persons, according to research from the University of Alabama, with exceptionally low injury rates that are consistent across all ages and intensities.

2. Enhances bone density

The body breaks down old bone and replaces it with new bone tissue to maintain healthy bones, however, beyond age 30, bone mass stops growing.

You gradually start making less bone than you are losing in your 40s and 50s. Exercise helps prevent osteoporosis, a condition that weakens bone and raises the chance of breakage as you age, by helping you build bone density while you're younger.

According to the National Osteoporosis Foundation, osteoporosis, which costs the healthcare system $19 billion annually, puts almost half of all persons aged 50 and older in danger of fracturing a bone. Nonetheless, conducting weight-bearing activities throughout one's life helps develop bone mass and strength, so this does not imply that elderly people are helpless.

Exercises like walking or aerobics are particularly crucial after menopause since osteoporosis affects women more often than it does men. Physical exercise may help stop bone loss when the elderly are unable to increase their bone mass. Cycling, yoga, and swimming are examples of low-impact workouts that may assist to improve balance and lower the risk of falls and fractures but are insufficient to slow bone loss.

3. Telomeres may become longer with exercise.

Telomeres, which resemble the caps on shoelaces, are the caps at the ends of DNA strands. As they become older, their length shortens, which adds to cell senescence, which causes the cells to stop dividing. Telomere length is associated with several chronic diseases, including heart disease, stroke, and high blood pressure. Compared to persons who are sedentary, research has shown that greater levels of physical activity are associated with longer telomere lengths in certain individuals. The elderly appear to be particularly susceptible to this. It is currently unclear if this association is causative, and several other factors probably influence telomere length. However, it is thought that having longer telomeres lowers the likelihood of developing age-related disorders.

4. It may raise mental capacity.
According to the National Institute on Aging, being able to switch between activities rapidly, organize an activity, and reject extraneous information are all indications of excellent cognitive function.
One of the most effective ways to maintain cognitive function throughout life and lower the

risk of age-related cognitive decline is currently thought to be physical exercise. Although it is still unclear if exercise may help prevent dementia, studies have shown a correlation between increased physical activity and a lower incidence of dementia, including Alzheimer's disease.

As scientists continue to study the impacts of exercise, they are discovering a variety of fascinating advantages. For example, working out your muscles releases myokines, which are tiny chemicals that have several advantages for your brain. It is also a great technique to increase the quality of your sleep, which is important since we know that sleep quality affects health quality.

We still don't fully understand how exercise impacts aging, but we do know the following: exercising your body Moving more often is preferable than moving less frequently—five times a week, for at least 30 minutes each day. You don't have to exercise continuously; it builds up over time (but, check with your health provider before starting any new activity).

Yet for the majority of individuals, a mix of aerobic and resistance training seems to provide the most advantages. The best part is that you can always start now.

CHAPTER 4

Five Strategies To Reduce Stress And Benefit Your Heart

Controlling unhealthy behaviors and relaxation is essential for heart improvement.

Persistent stress may have significant physical impacts on the body, whether it comes from a congested daily commute, an unpleasant marriage, or a demanding workplace. It is connected to a variety of health concerns, including mood, sleep, eating disorders, and heart disease.

The specific effects of persistent stress on the heart are unknown to medical professionals. While it has not been confirmed, stress most certainly causes inflammation, a recognized heart disease initiator. The prevalent wisdom, in my view, is that stress is harmful to your heart, but the evidence is considerably murkier and stress may have a more subtle impact on heart disease. Some individuals do respond in ways that enhance their risk for heart disease when they are under stress. For instance, individuals who are under stress often overeat and lack the energy or time to exercise.

Stress might also cause us to engage in other heart-harming habits like smoking and drinking alcohol.

It takes learning how to manage stress and regulating harmful behaviors to break the relationship. You may do it by following these five simple techniques.

- **Keep upbeat.** Laughing has been shown to enhance "good" HDL cholesterol, decrease stress hormone levels, and reduce artery inflammation.
- **Meditate.** It has been shown that this method of inwardly directed meditation and deep breathing lowers heart disease risk factors including high blood pressure. Yoga and prayer, which are closely related to meditation, may both help the body and mind relax.
- **Exercise**. Your body produces mood-enhancing substances called endorphins whenever you engage in physical activity, such as walking or playing tennis.

Exercise not only relieves stress but also guards against heart disease by regulating blood pressure, enhancing cardiac muscle strength, and supporting a healthy weight.

- **Unplug.** As stress follows you everywhere, it is hard to avoid it. severe the chord. Ignore TV news and emails. Make time every day to disconnect from the outside world, even if it's only for 10 or 15 minutes.
- **Look for a place to relax.** You may take a much-needed vacation from the tensions in your life by doing something as simple as taking a warm bath, listening to music, or engaging in a beloved pastime.

Chapter 5

What to Eat to Promote Longevity and Health

The five dietary practices that a qualified nutritionist says may lengthen your life.

The majority of individuals want to live longer. However, achieving longevity also means leading a better life with increased mental and physical well-being, including the capacity for activity and independence. I've seen many individuals in their 70s, 80s, and beyond who are healthier than people half their age throughout my time as a registered dietitian. Although there is some hereditary influence, lifestyle influences are more important, and diet plays a large part in lifestyle. According to research cited in a 2016 review of the literature in the journal Immunity & Ageing, only 25% of a person's lifespan is impacted by genetics; the remaining 75% is our choice of living.

These are five dietary practices you may follow to lengthen your life and live each year to the fullest.

1. Eat your fruits and vegetables
Eating more vegetable produce is perhaps one of the most significant and beneficial habits you can form, even if you probably hear this a lot. Regrettably, the majority of Americans are mistaken. Just around one in ten persons in the United States, according to the Centers for Disease Control and Prevention (CDC), consume enough fruits and vegetables. Just 10% of people meet the daily goal of two to three cups of vegetables, and 12% meet the daily goal of one and a half to two cups of fruit. Besides increasing your food intake, achieving those minimums may lengthen your life by years. A 2017 meta-analysis indicated that eating more fruits and vegetables is linked to a decreased risk of death from all causes, including heart disease and cancer. This finding was reported in the International Journal of Epidemiology. You should consider five servings or more each day.

More is good, but according to some studies, going above this point did not further lessen the chance of mortality.

How to Increase Fruit and Vegetable Intake

Include three cups of vegetables and two cups of fruit each day; one cup is equal to a tennis ball in size. Some advice: Try to establish a practice of eating a cup of fruit at breakfast each day and a second cup as part of a snack. Include one cup of vegetables for lunch and two cups for supper. Maybe mix the two. Two are eliminated by a smoothie that is created with a cup of frozen berries and a handful of greens. Entree salads and stir-fry dishes may also include fresh fruit, such as sliced apples or oranges.

2. Nuts and nut butter will drive you crazy

Nuts are a powerhouse of nourishment. They include essential minerals like potassium and magnesium, healthy fat, plant protein, fiber, antioxidants, and vitamins. It seems correct to say that they are related to life extension.

The metabolic syndrome, also known as insulin resistance syndrome, is a collection of illnesses that raises a person's risk of developing heart disease, diabetes, and stroke, according to the National Heart, Lung, and Blood Institute (NHLBI). The Journal of Nutrition released the results of a broader research which includes a randomized trial in 2020, that tracked 5,800 men and women with metabolic syndrome for a year. The findings imply that several metabolic syndrome indicators were reduced as nut intake rose. These indicators include weight, BMI, systolic blood pressure, waist circumference, and triglyceride levels. The good cholesterol HDL rose in the study in the female participants (but not the men).

Tips for Eating More Nuts
Two tablespoons of nut butter also qualify as a serving; an ounce of nuts equates to around one-fourth cup. Use nut butter as a dip for fresh fruit or celery, whirl it into your smoothie, mix it into oatmeal, or spread it over toast. Nuts may be eaten on their own or combined with salads, sautéed vegetables, and stir-fried dishes.

To coat fish or garnish foods like mashed cauliflower or lentil soup, crushed almonds work just as well as bread crumbs. Another fantastic approach to increase your intake is by baking with nut flours or using them in pancakes.

3. The Nuts Your Body Should Eat
Take More Meatless Meals
Mondays without meat have been a thing for a long time.

That's great, but for longevity, you should include plant-based meals in your diet more often than once a week.

The five regions in the globe where people live the longest, healthiest lives are described in a 2016 article in the American Journal of Lifestyle Medicine. These locations, known as the Blue Zones, may be found in different places, including Okinawa, Japan, and Ikaria, Greece. They all eat predominantly plant-based diets, which is one thing they have in common. Meat is consumed on average five times a month in portions of three to four ounces, or roughly the size of a deck of cards, while beans and lentils serve as the mainstays.

California's Loma Linda, which has the greatest percentage of Seventh-Day Adventists, is home to the sole Blue Zone in the US. This community, which is distinguished by its mostly plant-based diet, has an average lifespan that is ten years longer than those in North America.

For instance, a 2013 research from JAMA Internal Medicine compared vegetarians to omnivores and discovered that they had a considerably reduced chance of dying overall. The study included almost 73,000 Seventh-Day Adventist men and women. These comprised pesco vegetarians, lacto-ovo vegetarians (who do consume dairy and eggs), and vegans (who do eat seafood). Compared to the diet of non-vegetarians, vegetarian diets were linked with considerably reduced levels of cardiovascular disease risk factors, according to a 2019 follow-up research to 2013 one, published in the Journal of Nutritional Science. Researchers also examined the impact of dietary decisions on life expectancy in a 2022 study published in PLOS Medicine.

According to their findings, eating more whole grains, nuts, and legumes while consuming less red and processed meat would result in the greatest increases in lifespan.

How to Consume Less Meat
Replace meat in meals with pulses, which are a collective word for beans, lentils, peas, and chickpeas, to enjoy the advantages. Instead of adding chicken to a salad, have a side of lentil or black bean soup. To replace the meat in a stir fry, use black-eyed peas, and instead of jerky, nibble on vegetables with hummus. Investigate the ethnic eateries in your neighborhood that provide meals with pulses, such as Ethiopian lentil stew and Indian chickpea curry.

4. A Mediterranean-style diet
The most important aspect of eating for longevity is the general eating pattern, not any one food or food category. One of the best ways to live longer and in better health is to follow a Mediterranean diet.

The predominant food groups in this pattern include fruits and vegetables, whole grains, legumes, and healthy fats like avocado, olive oil, nuts, herbs, and spices. A couple of times every week, seafood is included. Along with limiting the intake of meat and sweets, the Mediterranean diet also allows for modest dairy, egg, and wine consumption.

Telomere length is a cellular-level lifespan indicator that is often mentioned in studies. Telomeres, to put it simply, are caps that guard DNA at the ends of chromosomes. A cell ages or becomes dysfunctional when they are too short. For this reason, shorter telomeres are linked to a decreased life expectancy and a higher chance of contracting chronic illnesses. Greater adherence to a Mediterranean diet may increase lifespan by preserving longer telomere length, according to research published in 2017 in the journal Oncotarget. According to the same research, the likelihood of dying from any cause decreases by 4 to 7% for every point raised on the Mediterranean diet scale (which gauges adherence to the diet).

A Guide to the Mediterranean Diet
You can swap butter for the nut or avocado butter on toast and extra virgin olive oil for sautéing veggies. Maintain simple meals and munch on fresh fruit with almonds, olives, or roasted chickpeas as a snack. With roasted potatoes or quinoa on the side, fish served over a bed of greens dressed in extra virgin olive oil, and a bottle of pinot noir, a meal following the Mediterranean diet may be considered balanced.

5. Which Foods Are Best and Worst for Your Teeth?

consume green tea:
Green tea is what I like to think of as preventive medicine in a cup. It has been associated in several studies with a decreased risk of obesity, type 2 diabetes, Alzheimer's, cancer, heart disease, and several other diseases. The greatest green tea consumers had reduced rates of cardiovascular disease and a decreased chance of dying from heart disease and stroke, according to a 2022 review of the literature that was published in the journal Nutrients.

There does seem to be some correlation between longevity and green tea consumption, even if it cannot be proven with certainty that drinking green tea will extend your life.

How to Consume More Green Tea
Green tea may be used to steam vegetables or whole-grain rice in addition to being sipped. It can also be used as the liquid in smoothies, porridge, or overnight oats. Moreover, it may be used in marinades, soups, stews, sauces, and marinades. Green tea that has been ground into matcha may also be used to make drinks and recipes. To avoid affecting the quantity or quality of your sleep, be sure to stop consuming any coffee at least six hours before bed.

A Brief Overview
It's the usual suspect when it comes to what to avoid doing. Avoid overeating and excessive sugar, processed food, meat, and alcohol intake. The good news is that the anti-aging foods listed above may quickly replace the anti-aging meals. Instead of manufactured cookies, choose an apple with almond butter, and choose green tea instead of soda.

In other words, if you concentrate on what to eat, you'll inevitably limit your consumption of items to avoid. That's significant because continuity is essential for longevity. Long-term nutrition promotes a long, healthy life!

CHAPTER 6

NINE VITAMINS AND MINERALS YOU SHOULD TAKE DAILY

As a child, do you recall eating those Flintstone vitamins?

The necessary daily supply of vitamins and minerals that you need for a healthy body may be obtained via supplements. Although eating a healthy, well-balanced meal is the best way to receive your vitamins and minerals, supplements may help your body.

In our bodies, vitamins have supporting functions to perform. Vitamins are necessary for the body to operate and to assist break down macronutrients like fat, protein, and carbs.

We outline the vitamins and minerals you need to consume daily along with their advantages.

Which vitamins should you take every day?

Around half of the American people are thought to take a vitamin or mineral supplement. Individuals may take supplements if they are aware that they are deficient in a certain food category. Others may do so because of the antioxidant advantages or because they are aware that they do not consume enough fruits and vegetables. Some folks could be lacking something.

Before beginning to take supplements, it is a good idea to speak with your doctor or a qualified dietitian since everyone has different vitamin requirements. They can assist you in determining which items to use or if you need to use any at all. If a supplement interacts poorly with any drugs you are already taking, it may result in health issues. Your doctor and pharmacist may advise you on this as well.

How much is a suggested daily allowance?
The average daily consumption of vitamins and minerals that a person requires to maintain good health and prevent deficiencies is known as the recommended daily allowance (RDA).

Vitamin and mineral requirements for men and women often vary.
The RDA may be measured in several ways. The body requires more of the vitamins and minerals that are measured in milligrams than those that are measured in micrograms. One milligram contains 1,000 micrograms. There is a defined RDA for each vitamin and mineral.

Many advantages of vitamins
These are the vitamins and minerals that you need to think about consuming.

A vitamin
Retinol is another name for vitamin A, a fat-soluble vitamin.
For women, the RDA for vitamin A is 700 micrograms, whereas for males it is 900 micrograms. Several dairy products and foods with yellow or orange coloring include vitamin A.
Good choices include apricots, mangoes, and cantaloupe.

The advantages of vitamin A
Assists by preventing infection
and sustains sound vision.
has a significant impact on kidney, lung, and
heart function.
maintains healthy skin by warding against
toxins (also called free radicals).
strengthens teeth and bones.

B vitamin
The vitamin B complex is made up of eight B
vitamins, each having a different RDA. The
United States Department of Agriculture
(USDA) reports that the majority of people do
not consume enough B vitamins each day to
meet the RDA.
To reduce the danger of deficiency, numerous
cereals, flours, loaves of bread, and portions of
pasta are regularly fortified in the United States
with B vitamins. B vitamins may be found in
whole grains, animal proteins, and leafy green
vegetables.
The bulk of B vitamins is crucial for converting
food into energy and are also crucial for cell
growth, development, and formation.

The advantages of vitamin B

keeps memory and brain activity at a normal range.
required for healthy protein, lipid, and carbohydrate metabolism.
lowers LDL (bad cholesterol) and raises HDL to reduce cholesterol (good cholesterol).
reduces the risk of heart failure and disease.
lowers the chance of a stroke.
essential for a healthy neurological system and blood cell synthesis.

C vitamin

Antioxidants included in vitamin C, a water-soluble vitamin, support the formation of healthy tissues. The RDA for males is 90 milligrams, while the RDA for women is 75 mg. A wide variety of fruits and vegetables contain vitamin C.

In addition to aiding in the production of collagen in your body, vitamin C helps shield your cells from the harm that free radicals may do.

The advantages of vitamin C
may lower the chance of contracting the common cold.
protects the health of the tissues and skin.
strengthens teeth and bones.
If you lack iron, vitamin C may improve your body's ability to absorb it. "More vitamin C is helpful if you're wanting to enhance your iron absorption," she continues.

Nutrition D
Ultraviolet (UV) light activates vitamin D, a necessary fat-soluble vitamin. Vitamin D is also present in cod liver oil, fatty fish, fortified drinks, milk, and cereals in addition to being obtained by sun exposure. When a person does not get enough UV light, they might be a healthy alternative. The RDA for both adults and children is 15 micrograms (600 IU). It is 20 micrograms for those aged 70 and older (800 IU).
Vitamin D deficiency is rather typical.
Your vitamin D levels may be checked by your doctor, and sometimes they may be so low that a prescription-strength vitamin D treatment is required.

The advantages of vitamin D
affects immune cell performance.
keeps the nervous system functioning.
necessary for healthy bones.
controls the calcium and phosphorus levels in
the blood.

Vitamin E
Vitamin E is crucial for maintaining the health
of your organs. Daily intake should be 15
milligrams. Vegetable oils, avocados, spinach,
seeds & nuts, and whole grains are sources of
vitamin E.
Vitamin E may aid in dilating blood arteries
and preventing blood clots in addition to its
antioxidant advantages in maintaining a robust
immune system

.

Benefits of vitamin E:
- Prevents poisons from damaging cells.
- keeps muscles functioning.
- lowers cancer risk.
- reduces the risk of heart failure and disease.
- decreases the chance of getting Alzheimer's.

Vitamins K

To help blood clot, vitamin K is necessary. Men need 120 micrograms of vitamin K daily, while women need 90 micrograms. The majority of this vitamin's protein-rich food sources are leafy green vegetables.
Along with calcium, vitamin K helps maintain your bones in top condition.

Benefits of vitamin K:
Promotes quick wound healing.
makes bones strong.
reduces the risk of heart disease.

Calcium

Calcium is a mineral required for strong bone development. The recommended daily allowance (RDA) for calcium is 1,000 milligrams for men and women aged 19 to 51; it rises to 1,200 milligrams for women aged 51 and older and men aged 70 and older (but be cautious not to acquire too much of it!). The majority of dairy products, including milk, cheese, and yogurt, as well as tofu, spinach, soy, and rhubarb, are rich sources of calcium.

Yet, it also affects how muscles work and is required for nerves to transmit signals from the brain to the body.

The advantages of calcium

enhance muscular performance.

aids in maintaining healthy blood pressure.

aids in the production of hormones.

helps to keep bones strong.

aids in maintaining healthy teeth.

reduces the chance of osteoporosis.

Iron

In blood, iron aids in oxygen delivery. A weakened immune system and exhaustion may be caused by a lack of iron.

The recommended daily iron intake for both sexes is 8 to 18 mg. Red meat, leafy green vegetables, and legumes are all sources of iron. Although there are many plant-based sources of iron, you simply don't absorb it as effectively, thus everyone who follows a vegetarian or vegan diet is at risk for developing an iron deficiency. Iron may be blocked by the quantity of fiber in a vegetarian or vegan diet.

The advantages of iron
- enhance immunological performance.
- offers energy.
- enhances brain activity.
- increases the capacity to concentrate more and stay alert.
- provides the blood with oxygen.

Zinc

Just trace levels of zinc are required. The RDA is 8 milligrams for women and 11 milligrams for males. In addition to beans, nuts, and whole grains, zinc-rich foods include red meat, poultry, and chicken.

Your immune system is strengthened by zinc, which may also help stave against infections like pneumonia.

Zinc benefits include
- lowering the risk of cancer.
- enhances the immunological system.
- enhances memory.
- reduces symptoms of the common cold.

Buying vitamins
The U.S. Food & Drug Administration (FDA) and the USDA do not regulate supplements. How can you determine whether the supplements you're buying are safe?
It is advised that you carry out the following before purchasing:

Speak with your doctor; Consult your doctor before adding any supplements to ensure that you need them and that they won't conflict with any prescriptions.

Check for independent testing; Some businesses submit their goods to a third party for independent ingredient verification.

Search for the USP logo; Supplying safe, high-quality goods is the mission of the independent, nonprofit United States Pharmacopeia (USP).

Think about the components; Stick to the fundamentals. Additions to vitamins' contents or claims are unnecessary and may have negative

consequences. Hence, even if supplements might be beneficial, pay attention to your diet and what you consume. Avoid substituting supplements for a balanced diet.

CHAPTER 7

RESEARCH ON AGING AND THE WAY FORWARD

Some people associate the term aging with fairness, knowledge, and advancement; others associate it with ugliness, illness, and demise. Aging now has a complicated connotation for me. When I was a young kid, I can recall counting my heartbeats while awake in bed, as though the beating in my chest mirrored the ticking of my biological clock. I assumed that a set number of heartbeats were allotted to each individual during their lifespan. As a young person, I consider aging as the gradual and inevitable countdown of these few heartbeats. While few would acknowledge it, the dread of getting older and dying is widespread. Our preoccupation with death has caused faiths and stories to grow and spread throughout history. Since then, scientific investigation has started to provide answers to one of life's biggest mysteries.

Historical Research on Aging

Alchemy was a thriving profession in the late Middle Ages. Obtaining the legendary philosopher's stone, which may give its user infinite life, was considered the holy grail of alchemy. There are no records of any successful attempts to synthesize the item despite several trials. There were other supposed anti-aging items besides the philosopher's stone. The idea of finding the elixir of youth in an unexplored continent grew in popularity after the discovery of the Americas. Juan Ponce de León, a conqueror, embarked on an unsuccessful search for the mythical spring in 1513.

The interest in "anti-aging science" and the attendant beliefs waned during the next decades.
Until James Birren developed a hypothesis combining what he termed the "tertiary, secondary, and fundamental phases of aging" in the 1940s, aging research was not well known.
 Gerontology, or the study of aging, was created by Birren, who also enlarged it socially and scientifically.

During the period, anti-aging therapies promoted by charlatans included dubious blood and serum infusions, which contributed to the designation of aging research as a pseudoscience. Oddly, recent research found that older mice that had plasma transfusions from younger mice had biologically better bodies, however, this hasn't been confirmed in humans and it's very obvious that the findings weren't known in the early 1900s. Scientists were drawn to this new and developing area of study thanks to Birren's leadership, and the stigma associated with aging in science started to fade.

There are still homologous analogous in humans. Research on life extension therapies has recently been concentrated on more sophisticated model species such as D. melanogaster, lab mice, and Rhesus monkeys. Several molecular processes have recently been linked to aging.

They include rapamycin, sirtuins, and reservatrol.

Reservatrol, a substance often present in red wines, stimulates sirtuin deacetylases, extending the lives of lower organisms and maybe contributing to human aging. Also linked to cardioprotective advantages is reservatrol. Pioneers like Harvard Medical School's David Sinclair have been at the forefront of the study of these systems and their links to aging. Mice have lived longer thanks to immunosuppressant therapy with rapamycin. An ongoing and promising area of aging research is the hunt for underlying molecular causes of aging.

The development of computer techniques for large-scale data analysis in the last ten years has uncovered exciting new information on aging. The quest for aging-related biomarkers has been accelerated by computational biology and bioinformatics.

The gold standards for biological age estimation in the past have been pulse wave velocity and telomere length, although, they only fully described a small portion of individual variation in aging.

Many physical and mental features, genetic abnormalities, and cardiovascular traits have all been linked in a recent study as possible biomarkers. A technique for estimating biological age (DNAm) using DNA methylation patterns was discovered in 2014 by UCLA professor Steve Horvath. It was significantly connected with chronological age and seemed to explain various trends in both aging and illness.

The main physiological mechanisms of aging are explained by a central aging signal, which is the subject of continuing study.

The public's attention to aging research has increased significantly during the last several years. The founder of the SENS organization and former computer scientist Aubrey de Grey presented a plan for overcoming the problem of aging in a very well-received TED presentation. The plan divides the aging process into four main categories: **aggregates, cross-linkage, cellular senescence and growth, and mutations**.

The issue can be managed more effectively and there is a chance that human life might be extended gradually over many years of medical developments if each sector is targeted independently. The possibility of anti-aging remedies has been emphasized by other social movements like transhumanism.
Emerging technologies are welcomed by transhumanism because of their potential to improve human health or quality of life, including extending healthy life spans.

Controversies
The aging study has been a contentious area since the time of alchemy. The advancements in aging research and rejuvenation technologies now raise two main concerns. First, those opposed to anti-aging science are worried about the real prospect of population growth. A micro-example of what an ageless population would look like is the age distribution of the population in the United States now. There are already worries that the Baby Boomer generation's aging population may put too much strain on the healthcare and Social Security systems.

Imagine the same result, but with the older end of the age range being added continuously and cumulatively.

Yet many who hold this view do not evaluate what the latest findings in aging science mean for potential anti-aging treatments. Almost all recent research in model organisms has shown that anti-aging medications tend to encourage prolonged, healthy aging. In other words, the relative ages of people would only be dispersed across a wider time frame. Those who are receiving therapy yet are 70 years old physiologically maybe 50 years old. As a result, in a relative world, concerns about a population skewing toward the elderly are mostly unjustified. A person would be more productive throughout their lifespan if they lived longer, healthier lives.

Religious and ethical objections are raised by some detractors of aging research. After all, are we not playing God if we are prolonging our lives beyond what is naturally possible? There is no easy way to solve these problems.

Scientists should be aware of these ethical considerations as they continue to conduct this field of study since there will always be supporters and opponents of aging research. If an anti-aging therapy is obtained, it is merely an extra opportunity that has been prolonged and is in no way required.

The Way Forward
These studies highlight the advantages of thoroughly analyzing medical interventions, risk factors, and drugs utilized in clinical practice. Do you anticipate similarly exciting advancements in the field of new therapeutics? In reality, I can offer you instances of how more molecular knowledge is already being used for potentially fruitful therapies.
The role of mitochondria, the energy-producing organelles in cells, has undergone several modifications related to the so-called pillars of aging, the elements of the developing area of geroscience.

Studies using experimental models have shown that strategies for maintaining or enhancing mitochondrial activity during aging affect results and health. These results are now being included in preliminary studies.

Cellular senescence is another illustration that has gained a lot of attention recently.

Just recently, we believed that cells were immortal. Today, we are aware that this is untrue. Senescence was first used to refer to replicative senescence, which is when cells stop dividing. We now know that a lot more things take place. Senescent cells don't just sit still; they produce a lot of inflammatory proteins as part of their aberrant phenotype.

Animal models used in genetic alteration experiments have produced some quite remarkable findings. The tiny number of senescent cells that are typically present in an experimental animal may be selectively eliminated by certain genetic changes.

Its musculoskeletal stability, the muscular mass, stamina while running, cognitive capacity, and general life expectancy are all increased by doing this.

As a consequence, chemical treatments in animal models may destroy the protective mechanisms that senescent cells have that maintain them around. Nevertheless, those genetic methods cannot be used to directly eradicate senescent cells in humans. Similar results have been seen with drugs or medication combinations created from medicines utilized in cancer treatment plans or as anti-inflammatories. Test animals that get such medications and specifically destroy senescent cells live longer and have higher function preservation, including brain, cardiovascular, and musculoskeletal functions. Several of the medications being studied for their ability to inhibit senescent cells have recently entered clinical trials. While we are unsure of their effectiveness, they do show how fundamental science may be translated into practical applications.

It's also a fascinating illustration of how ubiquitous inflammatory proteins and their effects may be throughout the body. It seems that alterations in the immune response are becoming more often linked to aging-related illness. True?

As we age, our immune systems undergo several modifications. But, it is oversimplified to believe that, as our immune systems become less responsive and dampened. Immune system alterations are not neutral; they are particular to a person. COVID-19 serves as an example. In older individuals, the immune system may be less receptive to vaccinations and other immunizations, but it may also overreact to infections and cause unwarranted, protracted inflammation. The hyperinflammatory response to the viral infection has been related to the startlingly specific susceptibility of older persons to morbidity and death with the recent COVID pandemic.

However, COVID is teaching us more information about the impact illness may have on the elderly. They transcend mere infection. What has to be done to provide care for elderly persons who are institutionalized and have had their social networks altered? We are beginning to ask more of these questions. Increasing older folks' social engagement and connection to their healthcare system will be an important part of our caregiving approach.

It's critical to support and maintain the social, behavioral, and economic components of older people's lives and learn about the clinical aspects of immune system function in these individuals.

The study of aging is a fascinating and expanding area. Research in related fields like cancer, diabetes, and Alzheimer's is expected to gain more knowledge as our understanding of the basic aging process advances.

The current development of biotechnology and big data-supported research is beneficial for the still-relatively understudied subject of aging study. One might anticipate further advancement and innovation in aging studies in the next decades. One day, maybe, even the mythical philosopher's stone or youthful elixir may appear as a result of this drive for deeper understanding.

Chapter 8

Live long, be well: Science-based advice for healthy aging,

Although it is good to celebrate becoming older, however, taking care of your body, mind, relationships, and mental health is beneficial for your health at any age.
You may remain independent, happy, and healthy for years to come by following these scientifically proven methods.

Make a move
Exercise may improve mobility, lower the incidence of fractures and falls, and delay the onset of several aging-related disorders. Also, it may stimulate the brain, which can aid in activities like processing information, learning new things, paying attention, and problem-solving.
As you age, it's more crucial to engage in certain types of exercise:

Exercises that build heart and lung fitness and improve circulation, include swimming, bicycling, dance, and endurance sports.

Exercises that keep your muscles strong include weightlifting, resistance band training, and carrying groceries.

Tai chi and balancing on one foot are two balance exercises that may aid with coordination and strength-building to lower the risk of falls and fractures.

Yoga and other activities that increase flexibility may keep you limber and prevent injuries.
The amount of physical activity recommended by experts each week is 2.5 hours or a little over 21 minutes each day.

Eat well. A diet rich in vitamins, minerals, and nutrients maintains your body and brain healthy and may lower your chance of developing certain aging-related disorders.
Give nutrient-dense foods a priority, including lean (low-fat) meats and poultry, plant-based proteins like nuts and seeds, and seafood.

Reduce your intake of foods that include harmful ingredients like extra sugar and saturated fat.

Accept fruits and veggies, please. According to research, consuming five servings of fruits and vegetables each day might lower your chance of developing certain chronic illnesses.

Watch how much you eat. Keep track of how much you consume and consult your doctor about the number of calories that are ideal for your lifestyle and diet.

One example of a diet that's excellent for heart health and may enhance the brain's capacity for thought and memory is a Mediterranean-style diet, which contains nuts, vegetables, and seafood.

Put your physical wellness first. Little adjustments add up. Start now for longer-lasting health advantages.

Don't drink as much. Drinking may exacerbate health issues, particularly as you age. If you drink, consider limiting yourself to one drink per day or fewer, or give up alcohol entirely.

Putting sleep first. Try to get between seven and nine hours each night. Establishing a regular sleep schedule and a nighttime ritual helps promote healthy sleep hygiene.

Stop using tobacco and smoking. Even if you have smoked for a long time, giving up the habit today can make you feel better straight away and might add years to your life.
Continually monitor your health. Ensure that you get frequent checkups and that you are up to date on your immunizations and health tests.
Don't neglect your mental wellness.

Attempt to manage your tension.
Persistent stress may harm the body and brain, especially the regions of the brain responsible for memory and learning. You may control your

stress by using techniques like regular exercise, meditation, and social interaction with friends and family.

Be vocal if you're feeling sad. Do not be reluctant to seek help if you are experiencing mental health issues. Help is on hand!
Maintain your connections. Feeling lonely and socially isolated may be bad for your mental, emotional, and cognitive health at any age. You may feel more involved and connected if you establish and maintain strong social bonds.

Consider serving as a volunteer for a neighborhood group.
arranging for frequent check-ins with distant friends and relatives.
establishing connections with others in your neighborhood. Join a neighborhood group or get to know your neighbors.

Use your brain. Almost as vital as physical exercise is a mental exercise. Regularly challenging mental exercises keep the mind busy and healthy and may delay the onset of cognitive loss as you age.

Try Picking up a new hobby, skill, language, or game.
Going out and about—you may attempt an exercise class or visit a museum pursuing your interests, such as reading a book, playing the guitar, or preparing a healthy dinner.

Join a research study
To encourage health, happiness, and good aging throughout life, scientists are always discovering new facts about the aging process. A fantastic method to advance science and better lives is to take part in clinical research studies. Learn more about clinical research and how to participate in studies as a volunteer.